THE GOLDEN SANDALS

Greg Bauder

Greg Bauder

All rights reserved, no part of this publication may be reproduced by any means, electronic, mechanical photocopying, documentary, film or in any other format without prior written permission of the publisher.

>　　Published by
>　　Chipmunkapublishing
>　　PO Box 6872
>　　Brentwood
>　　Essex CM13 1ZT
>　　United Kingdom

http://www.chipmunkapublishing.com

Copyright © Greg Bauder 2008

Edited by Katie Davey-Williams

Chipmunkapublishing gratefully acknowledges the support of Arts Council England.

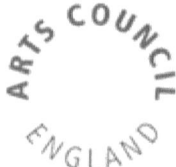

THE GOLDEN SANDALS

Chapter 1

Zen, who was only nine, sat in the desert resting his blistering feet under the two suns' heat. He had become lost from his nomad tribe after a sandstorm for some time now - and without his sandals. Night was falling on the desert and he was scared, so he prayed to OULI, his tribe's God to save him. He waited as the five moons rose in the sky, casting shadows. He was trying not to cry, as he closed his eyes and rested on a warm sand dune. He fell asleep, dreaming of his father.

Zen found his father in the desert but he felt strange because his dad seemed different. They were walking the stony, cracked desert to the market. They saw an eagle rise into the sky with two fish in its beak. Their eyes sparkled with wonder, like sunshine on waves where they themselves had just caught two silver fish. The eagle would be thankful, just as Zen was to be back with his father. They had taken two salmon out of the mighty west coast river, The Fraser.

Zen and his father approached the bread man at the market, and saw this dough-white grocer wave on the west street-side at them. Feeding people through trade was the way the desert people survived.

"We need to stop at the bread-grocer to get some bread," Zen's father said. It was strange how his father's dark skin had a gold-like shine to it.

"Hello, Joe," the grocer smiled, "I see you've brought along little B.J.
Hello B.J."

"Hello," answered B.J. smiling. His teeth were as white as camel bones; his hair was ebony. Zen wondered how the grocer knew his nickname, B.J. He thought only his parents called him that.

Zen's father bought five loaves of bread, and

THE GOLDEN SANDALS

the grocer piled them into the basket while joking that the whole Unknown Desert could be fed with that much bread. The two of them began the walk home. Zen's father said they would take a different path up the sand hill to their tribe.

"On the way, I'll show you a wishing well."

Zen was very curious, "What's that, Dad?"

"You'll see." He patted his son's head. Then, they saw a ragged man tipping over a garbage bin in an alley behind the market, looking for food. Zen and his dad walked in slow silence for half an hour.

Suddenly, from a thorny bush crowned with blood-red roses, a magnificent white dove rose through the sky with an olive branch. It flew, and Zen's eyes got sore watching its heavenly landing in its nest in a towering maple tree.

Greg Bauder

"Aren't doves beautiful birds?" Zen's father asked. "Oh! Here it is - the wishing well! "

The boy peered into the wishing well; it was spotted with gleaming coins. The coins' designs were hidden by the rotting fig leaves on top.

"Would you like to throw in a coin?" He asked his son.

"Yeah!" Zen responded, his eyes bouncing bright, like tiny emerald crystal balls.

"First you make a wish, though," he explained, giving the boy a golden coin.

"Okay, I wish for -"

"No, no. You don't tell me. It's supposed to be a secret, like when you blow out candles on a birthday cake."

THE GOLDEN SANDALS

"Oh," the boy said, pausing. Suddenly, he threw the gold coin into the pool, where it reminded him of a tiny, shiny and round noon sun. It was baptised, he thought, like the holy man had done to his tribe last year.

"Do wishes always come true here, Dad?" the boy asked, with a serious gaze.

"I would imagine so."

"What do they do with the money when they take it out of the well, Dad?"

"Well, they probably give it to charity."

"What's charity?" his son asked.

"Charity is when you help someone who is in need, like the poor or sick."

"Yeah?" the boy said his face purposeful with deep thought.

"What are you thinking about, B.J.?" his father asked him.

"About that man in the alley." The child hesitated. "Dad, can I have my allowance a day early?"

"Certainly, my son." His father unpocketed some coins and gave some to Zen. "Are you going to buy something?"

"Sort of!" And then he threw his entire allowance into the well.

His father smiled and said, "You're a good boy, Billy-John! And you're destined for great things."

Zen awoke in wonder. He was just

THE GOLDEN SANDALS

dreaming. And the cool night was now turning into a warm morning.

Chapter 2

Zen began walking and thinking about his strange dream. He wondered if the dream was really about him, since he had never heard of Billy-John. He suddenly found himself walking towards the same wishing well as in his dream. He got to the wishing well, but it disappeared in the heatwave. Zen knew it was a mirage and began to cry. He was nearly ready to give up because he knew he needed to walk, but his feet hurt so much.

Suddenly a little golden-robed genie appeared! Zen was uncertain whether the genie was real or a mirage, until the golden-turbanned little genie spoke, saying he would give him any golden thing he wished for. But only one wish, he added. Times are tough for all of us, he said to Zen. Even for mean people.

Zen couldn't put his aching feet out of his

THE GOLDEN SANDALS

thoughts, and with nothing to lose he decided to ask the tiny genie for a cool, new pair of golden sandals. In an instant the genie magically blessed Zen's feet with brand new golden sandals. Zen then thanked the disappearing little genie, whose whisper in Zen's ears said, "Beware the Shadowy Dragon."

Zen carefully began his journey again. His feet felt as snug as a rug in the sandals. After awhile, Zen rested and drank from his water container, which he kept in his cloak pocket. He was very surprised to find that he had drunk the last of his water. An hour later, his tongue was swollen dry by the suns. He began to cry as he walked, until he noticed a wishing well in the distance. Maybe he could fill his water container and get directions to go home, because there had to be people near a well. Maybe he would find his dad there!

As he neared the well, a little witch

appeared before him. She had on a sparkling silver witches' hat, with a golden robe and thin white slippers. The little witch told Zen that she knew he needed water. But he had to have something valuable that she needed, such as, some money to throw in the wishing well. Zen was sad again and asked the witch - whose name was Wondeau - if he could have some water for free, since he didn't have any money. Wondeau said she would like the golden sandals, and she asked him if he would give them to her for all the water he needed, forever. She said that with a little magic touch of her silver wand his water container would never be empty. He agreed, since his thirst was worse than his sore feet. The smiling little witch removed his sandals and handed him a map that said "Go west" on the top. Then she said to Zen, this was the way that she made a living, through trade. Wondeau was a divine water witch. Wondeau told him to follow the map.

Zen drank from the water container, and

THE GOLDEN SANDALS

thanked her. Then the nine-year-old boy, who had sold his golden sandals, walked the desert with nothing to lose. He began drinking his fill of water whenever he pleased, but his feet blistered beneath the suns and the desert sand. He took a look at the map and at the bottom of it was written, "sole washing". Then, Zen realized that he ought to wash his feet. The water streamed from his container, cooling his feet from the heat. Zen happily kept wetting his feet with water as he wandered the desert guided by Wondeau's directions, and he didn't miss the sandals.

After awhile, Zen rested at a sand dune, the first stop on Wondeau's map. But he was puzzled when he read, "Beware the giant shadow". Suddenly, Zen saw the head of a dragon's shadow! He turned to see a giant dragon, breathing fire at him from a hundred metres away. Zen's map read, "mouth wash". Quickly, he squeezed his magic canteen and the water jetted down the dragon's mouth. Soon the dragon fainted

Greg Bauder

and fell dead in the desert, its skin smoking.

THE GOLDEN SANDALS

Chapter 3

Zen then went west again and after the second cactus on the map, he saw an awesome scene. There was a group of people with white skin, dressed in golden clothes and all of them had golden sandals! These people must be wonderful, Zen felt, watching their caravans speeding about on four round wonder rocks. But what perfect rocks, he thought. He stared at the caravans for longer than he wanted, because suddenly a man was coming after him. Zen couldn't run as the man held Zen's arm and asked him what he was doing near here. Zen said he was lost, from the tribe of Bidah. The man seemed angry, and Zen became afraid.

The man ran rope over and over Zen's hands until Zen was unable to move them. He led Zen to the people in his tribe of Anerada. Their hair was a golden colour, which shone golden and long - even the young men's. The caravans had stopped and the people watched him being taken into what was a gigantic living tent, Zen thought. "OULI save me!" Zen called out, as he had seen the people of Bidah call out loud, when they knelt to pray.

The effect on the men was awesome when they heard him pray. They asked him if he had seen a genie in the desert that went by the holy name of OULI. Even at nine, Zen sensed that these people feared OULI and so Zen began to chant, asking for OULI. He felt a little surprised when the men left the tent, falling all over one another to escape. Zen left the tent and asked - actually he told the men - to remove the strings on his wrists. After a man released Zen's stinging wrists, Zen groped in his cloak for the map off Wondeau. It said to spray the golden people's skin with a piece of the map torn at the corner and dropped in his canteen. He did this as directed and the golden people fled. All but one.

Zen saw then that the child left behind had

THE GOLDEN SANDALS

silver hair and wasn't wearing sandals. She seemed to be about seven and she was very dirty. Her feet were blistered from the desert heat. Zen glanced at the map and folded it into his cloak. He knew what to do. He pressed a jet stream from his canteen, which cooled the poor child's feet. Zen felt glad at helping the little girl. Then, a whirling cloud of dust came about - and out of the warm sandstorm hopped Wondeau!

Wondeau hugged Zen like a friend and kissed the little girl's cheek. She stated to Zen that he had passed the test she had given him. With her wand, Wondeau gave the girl and Zen golden sandals. The girl's skin turned golden like Zen's and the divine water witch, Wondeau's. Then, Zen noticed the golden people being led home by a gigantic rope - by the genie he had seen first in the desert! But the golden people were no longer golden. Their hair was black and their skin dark. The genie freed them and let them go towards home. He was OULI, he said to Zen and the rest of the people.

Greg Bauder

Wondeau was his wife, OULI smiled. They waved and the mean people cried and said sorry.

THE GOLDEN SANDALS

Chapter 4

Zen felt in his heart that he had to leave. He began walking across the desert when he noticed Wondeau and the little girl following him. He was puzzled because of this. Turning, Zen called to the girl and Wondeau to come towards him. In a dazzle of light, they were beside him. Wondeau smiled at Zen, and asked him if he would help her and Goodwen battle King Jas and his shadowy dragons in a faraway part of the Unknown Desert. Zen said he would be glad to help them but asked if they could help him find his tribe afterwards. Wondeau nodded yes and beamed love. They began to walk towards King Jas' faraway castle. It was soon dark so they stopped and rested on the warm dunes. Zen was tired and fell asleep right away.

Zen, Wondeau and Goodwen stood before King Jas in a faraway place. King Jas had ordered his top scholars to translate some holy books from an ancient language. But strange stars had begun to appear in the sky above the King's city. The King was afraid of the night lights and wondered if they were signs from his god. The King had scarcely slept for three nights. King Jas welcomed them with a feast, and as they ate he asked the three of them if they knew why the stars hovered over his city.

Wondeau said it takes many years to learn the ways of wisdom and magic. The lights were signs of a new age dawning, where peace would guide the world and Kings would no longer cause wars. The King asked her how she knew these things. She said he wouldn't understand. The King did not like her secrecy and said if she didn't tell him she would be tried for heresy and witchcraft. Wondeau said the ways of love; wisdom and magic were not for fools. King Jas ordered his fool out. The three of them laughed, and the cowardly King had his guards throw them in his dungeon. It was dark in there until they saw a bright flame of

THE GOLDEN SANDALS

fire. The Shadowy Dragon! Zen became frightened and reached for his canteen, but instead Wondeau was holding him and saying it was just a dream. Then, Wondeau was hugging Goodwen who had also dreamed of King Jas. The three of them talked until it became clear that Zen and Goodwen had dreamed the same dream.

Chapter 5

The three of them left early in the morning and began walking across the desert sand. Zen was hungry and knew Wondeau and Goodwen were, too. Then, in the distance, Zen saw the market in the strange dream he had had about his father! The bread-grocer was the same pale man, and Zen nearly fainted when the man said, "Hello, B.J."

Wondeau smiled and Goodwen asked if there was a wishing well nearby. Zen was surprised. But, they needed food, so Zen offered his golden sandals. Wondeau said no and that the man could have her and Goodwen's golden sandals in a deal for bread. Zen told Wondeau he didn't understand why he couldn't help pay, but she said he would in other ways. When the time was right, she told him and she hugged him.

They got their bread and settled down by an

THE GOLDEN SANDALS

alley entrance. The three soon noticed a poor, ragged man going through garbage bins. Zen got up and picked up a loaf of bread and handed it to the man. The man turned into OULI.

"You are learning wisdom, Zen. Or should I say B.J.?" Wondeau said as she kissed OULI and told the children to rise.

Zen and Goodwen rose. OULI clapped his hands and a magic carpet appeared beneath their feet. Soon, they were rising above the desert until they got to the New Lands. When they arrived in the New Lands they were greeted in the natives' village with joy, since the elders could see that they were special and blessed.

Their high priestess, Sari Mara, was humble and she treated her friends with love and honour. Zen knew he must help her people, because Sari Mara told them her people did not like King Jas as he was a cruel ruler. And although Zen missed his family, he loved the New Lands people and the large, leafy cactus-like trees he had seldom seen. Around the village there were also many strange animals and bright plants.

Zen and Goodwen were allowed to wander close to the village but they had to be careful. They were becoming good friends and would laugh and play games with the other children. But, they were taught poetry everyday by Sari Mara. Zen began to love poetry and he graduated to the private teaching of Apphoe, a very wise and elderly woman. Apphoe greeted him one morning and beside her was a strange, beautiful woman. Apphoe said her time was almost over and the new woman, Jonark, would teach him how to help defeat King Jas. The next day Apphoe was gone.

Jonark began to tell Zen that he would soon learn many great secrets. She said he was a fast learner; Zen was so eager to understand things that he came to her with many questions. Then,

THE GOLDEN SANDALS

one day Jonark led Zen, Goodwen and Wondeau into an underground cave system with many men and women rebels. Zen and Goodwen were at first afraid of the cool, closed-in tunnels, but they became used to them.

Zen had always wondered what it was like under the ground. But, there was little time for Jonark was disappointed to learn that the scholars, who had helped her as a child escape, had all been charged with treason and that King Jas had imprisoned them. He had built up a powerful army to feel more secure, but Zen knew he was a coward and he almost pitied him. Jonark decided that Zen would defeat the King's swords.

The underground people began to write their views that Jonark and a boy named Zen would defeat King Jas. They said Zen was from a faraway world and was their prophet. When these writings were published, Zen was told that his golden sandals would allow him to meet those who no one else could face. Zen knew then why it was so important for him to have these sandals. They had saved him in the desert and now he was to be taken by a star over the lands of Jonark's friends to drop thousands of books and papers. Zen was very calm, even though he was about to meet strange beings. Soon the time was near and Jonark, Wondeau and Goodwen hugged him; then, he climbed the ladder out of the cave.

Zen saw that it was dark and cloudy, yet through the trees came a golden light. The light was an oval form and it landed beside him. Zen watched, fascinated but still calm, as a door to the light opened. Then he saw the strangest beings he had ever seen. They were small, grey alien males and females, with big heads and large dark eyes. They talked to him in his mind and explained to him that his golden sandals could create miracles.

Zen knew what he had to do. He clicked his sandals together until he turned into a giant. He

THE GOLDEN SANDALS

was about fifty meters tall and his canteen was heavy in his cloak pocket. He opened the tunnel door and with one hand he grabbed the boxes of books and writings of the underground people. He put them in the ship, then went back to his normal size and entered the ship that he had been told had come from another planet. Soon, with the aliens he began throwing the writings over King Jas' city, which was surrounded by a huge moat full of shadowy, fire-breathing dragons.

The people gathered them up and marvelled at the brilliant writings. All except for King Jas who knew that Jonark was a poet and a prophet. The King immediately announced a million sheckings reward for the head of the poet/priestess. The aliens taught Zen that Jonark could not defeat the King without Zen's special powers. Zen loved the aliens, which made him determined to succeed and help his friends. He got off the ship near the moat and clicked his golden sandals together, which again turned him into a giant. Strangely though, the moat had no water, but Zen soon saw it was full of fire-breathing dragons.

Zen reached for his canteen as the dragons began to spit fire. One by one he sprayed water down their throats until they were all destroyed, except for the largest dragon. This dragon galloped away screaming, "We will meet again!" Zen pocketed his giant canteen and returned to his normal size. He smiled with satisfaction when he saw the lights above the city. But, he still missed his family.

The next day, Jonark led her army towards the King's castle. Quickly, the King's knights deserted him after despising him for many years. There was barely any resistance by the King's forces; soon Jonark had control of the castle. When the war was over, King Jas jumped to his death from a tower. Jonark was voted Queen by the people. At her crowning, she announced that poets would be her legislators, but someday all

THE GOLDEN SANDALS

would learn and share equally in the magic of wisdom. Zen held Goodwen's hand and Wondeau promised that in about a dozen years they would be married. After the crowning of the queen, Zen went to a beautiful room in the castle and he fell asleep. Aliens whispered that he was about to enter a new life.

Chapter 6

Usually on Saturdays during winter in British Columbia, young Billy would be out having snowball fights, making snowmen or, if there wasn't enough snow, he would help his older brother build car models in their room. But this weekend, after dinner, Billy's father asked him if he'd like to watch the hockey game with him. It was his introduction into Hockey Night In Canada. The year was 1963.

Billy watched and listened to his father and the announcer with fascination, as they explained what was going on in the game. He didn't understand a lot of it, but he was thrilled when a guy named Stan scored a goal and his father, and the TV fans, cheered. Billy liked how the puck hit the back of the net, but he was impressed with the hockey sticks the most. It must be so much fun to whack a puck into the net, he thought.

THE GOLDEN SANDALS

Billy had seen older kids playing the game in the streets before, but he had never had an interest in hockey. Until now. Now he yearned to play - with a hockey stick of his own. All that night he dreamt about the sticks, pucks, numbers, nets - and practically everything else. He knew his goal was his very own hockey stick.

The next morning after breakfast, Billy's father took him, his two brothers and his two sisters, to the gas station to return some spark plugs. They all went inside with their father, and Billy saw the most desirable vision he could imagine - hockey sticks on sale for a dollar each! He asked his father for his monthly allowance a little early, but his father shook his head as Billy pleaded with him.

"You're already overdrawn at the Allowance Bank," he said to Billy. "Besides, if I give you a dollar then I have to give the others one, too." Billy was disappointed but somehow knew that he would get one of those almost magical sticks out of the barrel - but he was in a sticky situation. He had no money. He was shut-out.

When they got home Billy decided on a plan - he would earn the money. And since it had just snowed, he thought that he could make money shovelling walks like his older brother sometimes did. But he knew he wasn't strong enough for the job. Then he prayed to OULI to bring him his golden sandals. Like magic they were on his feet and he put his rubber boots on over them. He could feel their power and grinned. He got the snow shovel out of the garage and went next door to the elderly couple, the Smith's, who usually let Billy's older brother shovel the walk and driveway. At first they seemed rather doubtful about Billy's ability to do the job, but he begged them to let him at least try. Finally, they agreed.

It was a big task and Billy almost sweated hockey pucks doing it. But, he focused on those

THE GOLDEN SANDALS

gold, curved sticks protruding from the barrel in the gas station. His arms ached as he heaved the snow, but his heart ached more for a hockey stick. Finally, he finished and got a dollar-fifty from Mr. Smith who said he had done good work, even faster than his older brother, Burke. Mr. Smith said Billy was strong and would make a very good hockey player. Billy left feeling excited as he put the shovel back, and began the two block walk through the snow to the gas station. He got to the gas station and grabbed a golden, curved hockey stick from the barrel and paid for it. Then he began the walk home.

When Billy got home he went straight to the basement, where he picked up a rubber ball to shoot against the wall, like he had seen older kids do in the neighbourhood. He was all set to shoot the rubber ball when he sensed that something was wrong. His heart sank - he realized his stick curved the wrong way! He had bought a left-handed stick and he was right-handed! Shoot!

Tears began to form in his blue eyes as he dropped the stick, then a thought struck him: he would return the stick like his dad had just returned spark plugs that morning. He picked up the stick and put on his heavy winter coat. He left through the basement door and went back to the gas station. He was hopeful that the worker there would understand and he began to sweat in the freezing January weather. He entered through the gas station doors, which now seemed bigger. He approached the counter, his green eyes fighting back tears.

"What can I do for you, son?" asked the worker. "Did you pick the wrong stick?"

"Uh... yes...sir. I'm sorry."

"Well, it's okay, boy. It's happened before." Billy was relieved and thanked the man who helped him pick out a right-handed curved stick,

THE GOLDEN SANDALS

which was the right height as well. He thanked the friendly man again and eagerly left with his prize. Just the right stick!

Chapter 7

Zen woke in a strange bed. He was a little chilly and it was dark. He could hear snoring and through the window he saw Wondeau and Jonark. They held up his golden sandals and said the powers watching over him would help him through his new life. His new name was Billy and he would experience wonderful things on this new planet, and his golden sandals would be needed on sunny summer days there. Zen got up in the room and went to the window to watch his friends disappear. A voice behind him told him to go back to bed. It was his older brother, and he remembered a lot about his brother and family. But why was he here as Billy? He went back to bed and began to dream.

Zen grew up as Billy John Brighton. He was a small boy even for nine, and he liked to tag along with his older brother, Burke. Billy had gentle, green eyes and short, curly brown hair.

THE GOLDEN SANDALS

Unfortunately, he had a speech impediment that the older boys - including Burke - used to make fun of, but Billy would accept their insults because he loved his brother and wanted to be around the cool, older boys.

He liked to go hiking with Burke and his brother's two friends, Leroy and Jake, especially to the flats by the mile-wide Fraser River near the south of Vancouver. They liked to walk quickly through the busy streets and would laugh and say to Billy, who had trouble keeping up, "Fasther, Billy, fasther." Billy would feel weak and reply, "You shlow down." The boys would laugh again, but would slow down a bit for him. Today, Billy had sensed something was wrong, so he had worn his golden sandals.

They would reach the sandy, carpeted-like beach, and the older boys would grab a wooden raft and a long stick which they used as an oar. They never let Billy ride on a raft because he was too young, and even they would never paddle more than thirty feet from the shore of the mighty Fraser.

Billy would watch with admiration from the shore as his older brother and friends would have raft races and mock battles for "Pirate Captain". They would have sword fights with their oars and bump each other's rafts gently. Billy would sometimes sit on the log-boom reaching out from the shore so he could be closer to the action.

"Have you ever been to 'Shea', Billy?" they would say, making fun of his speech impediment, and howl with glee. Billy was four years younger than these boys, yet he knew by Burke's occasional wink that it was all in good fun. After the rafting and games were over Burke would buy each of them a Coke at the gas station, since he had a paper route and could easily afford it. Billy always felt special when Burke would hand him his Coke first after they were paid for. And he liked

THE GOLDEN SANDALS

it when the other boys asked him where he got his cool golden sandals.

Then, on Labour Day, the last day before school, Billy watched his brother and friends' usual antics on the "High Sheas" as they called it. They were out a little further this time, when suddenly a speedboat zoomed by close to them. Leroy fell awkwardly (as the speedboat vanished down the river) and struck his head on the edge of the log-boom Billy was on. Burke and Jake balanced their rafts like surfers.

Without hesitating, Billy grabbed Leroy by his collar and with all his strength he held him there. Billy was terrified when he saw Leroy's head was bleeding. Burke and Jake were soon there and told Billy to run to the gas station for help, whilst they began to pull Leroy out of the river.

"Please, go fast, Billy, fast," Burke said, frightened. The sand beneath Billy's golden sandals soon turned into cement as he approached the Petro-Canada gas station. His golden sandals had allowed him to run four blocks in ten seconds. He was out of breath as he told the gas attendants that an ambulance was needed for his friend. A worker inside phoned for one, while the gas attendant drove Billy down to the flats. The drive seemed to take forever. When they got there, the gas attendant checked the unconscious Leroy's breathing and covered him with a blanket, and wrapped a towel around his head.

    An ambulance arrived soon. The paramedics took Leroy away, after saying he would be okay. One of the paramedics said that if Billy hadn't acted so fast Leroy would have died.

    Billy was scared, but for the first time he felt a sense of pride despite his speech impediment. He wasn't just a dumb kid. He had saved a life! He watched the police arrive just as Burke said to

THE GOLDEN SANDALS

him, "You've been to sea, Billy, and nobody could have done it faster, Billy, nobody." These words from his beloved older brother made him glow with happiness, despite his concern for Leroy.

"You're okay, Billy," said Jake. The police questioned the boys, and then lectured them as they drove them home. The boys were never to go to the flats again, which was fine with Billy. He had only gone to feel like he was one of the guys. And now he was. Billy felt great when his brother thanked him again that night. But, Billy fell into a troubled sleep.

Chapter 8

Billy was lost in the wilderness as he tried to find his father's car so he could go back to their safe Vancouver hotel. Each tree seemed darker and more sinister as he swished through the leaves, the night descending before him. He heard a snap behind him. He dropped to his knees. He wished he hadn't gone to take a leak in the Fraser River so far from his fisherman father.

He heard that snap again and he rose up running. A tree branch hooked and ripped off part of his white tee-shirt; it occurred to him that his shirt was as bright as a beacon. He took it off and crumpling it into a baseball size, he threw it as far as he could. He could hear something breathing and rustling behind him, and then a hairy hand covered his mouth and he was shouldered and carried through thinning brush.
Whatever was carrying Billy was as strong as a bear. Billy was so shocked when they entered a

THE GOLDEN SANDALS

dimly lit cave that he blacked out.

He came to near the crackling glow of a fire circled by stones, piled eerily like a miniature Stonehenge that he had often seen on TV. He looked up to see ... he gasped... Bigfoot!

"Don't be afraid," he growled softly. "We will not harm you."

"Who are you?" Billy whispered hoarsely. He looked around the giant cave. Then a small, grey alien with big, black, hypnotic eyes came forth. Billy scrambled away, like a crab moving backwards.

"We are the watchers and guardians of this planet. We control the way this planet evolves. Do not be afraid, for you have been chosen to give this information when the time is right." He floated over the fire to Billy and placed his long fingers on Billy's forehead. Billy calmed down, immediately.

Greg Bauder

"But what about God?" Billy asked.

"You mean gods. You're looking at some. You see, we are all gods in the spirit world. Or heaven; or nirvana; or Elysium, as people on hell planets like yours calls it. Both rely on each other: the spirit world and your world interact and one day they will come together. You have been chosen by us to spread the word." Billy left the cave after learning more secrets and clicked his golden sandals together, to turn into a giant. He stepped over trees and saw his father's car in the distance. Then he went back to his normal size. He noticed strange lights in the sky as he saw his father.

"Father!" Billy screamed, as he sat up in his straw bed. "I had that same dream again!" He started to cry as he hugged his father, while his mother, Mary, lit a candle.

THE GOLDEN SANDALS

"Its terrible living here, Mary; we're getting out of here. To Egypt or India or both."

"Yes, Joseph. Let's go at dawn." He smiled at his parents and fell back into a deep sleep after they read from a holy book.

Chapter 9

Billy's mother, Mary, worked all day at a long-term care facility for the elderly. She was an exceptionally kind and caring person and could often understand the patients' needs before they did. Billy believed she had been given a special gift from their dog. But he never told anyone about his dog's ability to communicate his thoughts to him.

Mary would finish work at four PM weekdays and walk home to her waiting family and dog, Marvin. Marvin would telepathically tell Billy when she was approaching. She would smile and pat her beloved Springer spaniel, Marvin, when she entered the small green bungalow they owned. She would ask each child how school went, and then she would start dinner. One night after dinner, Billy was watching hockey with his Dad. Billy noticed that Marvin's ears suddenly moved and in a few seconds they could hear dogs

THE GOLDEN SANDALS

barking outside. He ran to the door, and telepathically told Billy that he wanted to check out the commotion. He was neutered, so there wasn't much danger of him fighting. He left, and ran down the street.

Billy had never seen him act this way. Several minutes later, there was a scratch at the door, and Billy opened the door to see a wide-eyed Marvin.

"There's danger where your mother works," he said in Billy's mind. "You must come - and hurry." Billy put on his golden sandals and went outside with Marvin, who telepathically pictured smoke. Billy knew there was a fire. He was so certain he picked up Marvin and ran the four blocks in about fifteen seconds, due to the power of his golden sandals. As they approached the facility, Marvin flashed the last room on his right paw side into Billy's mind.

Billy left Marvin outside the building and ran

inside. The staff asked him what he was doing there and that his mother wasn't working today. Billy was out of breath and said to check room A12 for smoke or fire. He ran by them and they followed in close pursuit. He touched the door handle and it was warm. He wondered why the sprinklers and alarm weren't working. Probably because it was an older building system, he thought.

"Get that fire extinguisher!" He said to a worker. They entered the room which was filled with smoke, and they saw in an instant what had happened as the worker doused the small fire. A young woman, who was a single mother of four, had been staying by her ill grandmother's side and had fallen asleep in her chair smoking. The woman had bags under her eyes, and Billy, despite his dislike of cigarettes, held her hands and guided her out of the smoke-filled room. The staff came out a few minutes later and said the woman's grand-mother was awake and the smoke

THE GOLDEN SANDALS

had not harmed her.

"But how did you know there was a fire here, Billy?" asked a young nurse.

"A friend who had passed by told me," said Billy who went out to see Marvin wink at him. They left the care centre's parking lot just as the firemen showed up. He rubbed Marvin's chin.

"You're a magic dog, Marvin," he said. He replied that Billy's golden sandals were the greatest magic. They went home.

Chapter 10

Zen remembered his dream about his father calling him B.J. He wondered why; as he lay in bed patting Marvin's head. No one on earth called him that. He fell into a deep sleep and was not surprised when Wondeau floated down from the heavens and told Zen to put his golden sandals on, as there was an emergency near Queen Jonark's castle. Zen waved goodbye to Marvin and followed the pretty little witch, Wondeau, out the window after he clicked his golden sandals. He could fly! The two landed in Egypt and went into a giant pyramid, which took them through a time portal to Zen's old world of the two suns and five moons.

They arrived in a dark land where a black cloud hung over Queen Jonark's castle. Surrounding the castle were pit bulls, an ogre and the giant dragon that had escaped Zen and who had said they'd meet again. Zen clicked his golden

THE GOLDEN SANDALS

sandals and was fifty metres tall again. Then Wondeau used her magic wand to create a gigantic hockey stick in his hands and a big puck at his feet. The ogre with one eye came towards him laughing, saying he'd have B.J. over for dinner. Zen let go a blazing slap shot with his stick, and the puck struck the ogre in the eye and killed him.

The giant dragon was furious. He then called his two hundred pit bulls from the moat to attack Zen, but Zen used the canteen in his pocket to jet spray them back into the moat until they drowned. The dragon roared and said he would not be stopped. He sent a breath of fire at Zen, who could barely hold it off even with his canteen at full power. So he dropped his canteen and let go a slap shot from his giant hockey stick and the puck struck the dragon between the eyes, knocking him over.

"Use your wisdom," Wondeau whispered to

Greg Bauder

Zen. The dragon rose and let go a frightening roar.

"I heard you, you fool," said the dragon. "Do you think playing hockey, saving people and having a telepathic dog makes you wise?" The dragon laughed. Zen knew then what he must do.

"I used my golden sandals selfishly, I admit, for the hockey stick since only I benefited from my plan. And I liked the attention I received when I saved Jake, when a true act of heroism is humility." Puffs of smoke were coming through the dragon's nostrils as the beast began to beg him to stop. "But, I learned from my loyal and magic dog, that true wisdom and charity are best served without a pat on the back. That is why we left before the firemen came. Now, they're going to have to cart you away." The dragon screamed and then exploded into tiny grey pieces. The clouds lifted and the two suns shone on Queen Jonark's city.

THE GOLDEN SANDALS

Chapter 11

Zen went into the city with Wondeau and Goodwen to meet Queen Jonark and their other friends. On either side of her were two familiar looking men. Zen introduced himself and his friends to the men but they told him they always had known him. They had lived on earth many times and he had been named after them. Zen said that they must be Billy and John. They smiled and said he was wise.
Billy spoke to Zen.

"My name was William Shakespeare on your planet. My friend, John, was John Milton. Your wise father named you after us." Zen said he had read their poetry when Apphoe and Jonark had been tutoring him in their words of wisdom classes, in the old village. They talked for several hours and enjoyed a great feast. Then, Goodwen approached Zen and said they needed to find her family. Zen and Goodwen said goodbye and told

THE GOLDEN SANDALS

them they were going back to their humble life as nomads, looking after sheep, cattle and camels. Zen and Goodwen set out that evening with Wondeau, and the two females were a little surprised when Zen told them to follow the star in the sky. It was a spaceship of the Gods' he said, and the three of them were thrilled and joyful. They walked all night and rested on a desert dune in the morning. Zen knew that it was easier walking at night because it was cooler. They went over dune after dune until late afternoon, when suddenly Zen cried out that he'd found his tribe!

His family hugged him and wondered who the young girl was. Suddenly, a man and woman came to Goodwen and thanked Zen for rescuing her from the mean people. They held her as their tears fell and the three retired to their tent. Zen's family asked him how he had managed to stay alive. Zen said, "Little people can be gifted."

Greg Bauder

THE GOLDEN SANDALS

THE GRAVITY GIRL by Greg Bauder

Chapter 1

Karla Wordsworth cried giant tears as she sat couched and cornered in the living-room. Her smile had disappeared with the tormenting window view, a view of summertime children in the neighbourhood, laughing, riding their bikes and playing. Chanel, her seven year old daughter, was no longer able to join in their fun because of a menacing shadow of illness that haunted the Wordsworth family. Karla rose, not even noticing that her cup of Red Rose tea had grown cold beside her as she decided to see if Chanel was feeling any better.

She could hear the children outside buzzing like bees as she hesitated in the hallway. New tears sprung from her eyes and she prayed inside for the millionth time for Chanel to be better. She had been fretting and terrified for months like the rest of her family, after seeking help for Chanel from baffled doctors. Karla didn't realize she had her back leaning against the hallway wall, as she agonized over her paralyzed child; a child who could no longer bathe or dress herself, or even chew food. She had to be strong for Chanel, so she went in the bathroom to pick up a towel. Her back ached as she reached for a towel. She knew it was from carrying Chanel so much.

    Karla dried her stressed, pallid face in the bathroom and struggled to put on a smile. Burt, her five year old son, came in just then and she asked "How's my boy?" He said he was sad because everyone was sad about Chanel. She gave him a hug and said the doctors would help Chanel. She patted his head and told him he could get a piece of her twelve year old daughter Anne's cake. He jetted off for the kitchen, as Karla, head held high though feeling low, entered the gloom of her

THE GOLDEN SANDALS

daughter's hellish room.

Karla panicked inside when Chanel did not even stir as she approached her bed.

"How's my punkin'?" she asked, trying not to let her voice break like a child's toy. When Chanel mumbled something, Karla's window shattered and she looked deep into her child's diamond-glazed eyes. She was frantic and knew she had to call her husband, Martin, at work. Anne came in just then and asked how Chanel was. Her face turned to horror as she saw the choking foam that was jutting out of Chanel's mouth.

"Call Dad, Anne," Karla whispered, as she held Chanel's hand. Anne flew out of the room for the phone. The doorway shadows on the walls danced like victorious snakes, but Karla knew they were symbols of her own fear from inside, and they'd be dashed to ashes when Chanel was better. She would fight for Chanel to the death in her God-forsaken world of love. She knew Martin, Anne and Burt was as traumatized as she was, but Chanel's condition was beyond comprehension, even to the doctors who had tested her for brain tumours and almost every other major illness.

"Suffer the little children to come unto Me," she found herself saying out loud, and suddenly Martin was there hugging her and asking how Chanel was. He then picked up Chanel after he saw her condition and carried her out to their van.

"Shouldn't we call an ambulance, Martin?" Karla asked, shaking beside the car.

"No doll, " he answered. "The hospital is close by and I'll watch Chanel, and she'll get there quicker this way."

"But -" Karla began, her face twisted with worry.

THE GOLDEN SANDALS

"Take Anne and Burt in and I'll phone you from the hospital." He kissed her, Anne and Burt; then reared out of the driveway and swung the van into the street. It was supper-time so there were no kids playing in the street, the street that Chanel had once run circles around. And now her illness, the enemy, had run circles under Chanel's eyes. And her green gills meant she may never play again on the green grass of home.

Karla turned to Anne and Burt, and they solemnly walked into their ghostly home. Karla sensed the terror they were undergoing so she said, "How about if we order pizza tonight?" She knew it was a weak attempt at a diversion, but she was relieved when Burt picked up a little. He was extremely bright, but she knew he was too young to fully understand the drastic grip that Chanel's terrifying disease had on her. But Karla knew Anne, who was mature and sensitive, was suffering from the petrifying cross that Chanel was bearing.

    Karla reassured Anne and Burt that Chanel would be fine and that she was getting the best of care at the hospital. Her stomach was a turmoil of horror as they all waited by the phone for news about Chanel. They all bore the panic of doom on their faces, and when the phone rang Karla grabbed it. It was the pizza place confirming their order. Karla restrained herself from swearing, but banged the phone down in frustration. She lit up a smoke and went to make a quick cup of tea from the microwave.

    She went back to the living room where Anne and Burt were floored watching TV. Then she gave Anne a twenty dollar bill from her purse to pay for the pizza; she knew Anne liked to do this, because Anne was very responsible. After Karla had smoked a few cigarettes and her tea, the pizza guy knocked and Anne paid for the pizza. Karla was only able to nibble at one piece, her

THE GOLDEN SANDALS

stomach in knots of despair. But Anne and Burt ate their fill, which she was glad for. Even their cat Missy had a few bites of pizza as Karla stretched out on the couch, hand by the phone, and then Missy sat on her lap. Karla asked Burt to turn on the living room light, as Karla thought the dying sunlight played wicked shadows on the walls.

Just as the horizon through the window melted the sun into night, the phone rang with a sharp, eerie, rattle. Karla answered it as they all prayed inward. It was Martin. When Karla's relieved and long-lost happy expression appeared, her two children's faces shone like new bicycles. She repeated her husbands' words that Chanel had been diagnosed and treated, and she was going to live. However, Chanel was being transferred to the Children's Hospital.

Karla repeated Chanel's ordeal as told by her husband, so Anne and Burt could share in the joyful news. Chanel had stopped breathing on the

way to the hospital. Martin had to pull over and clear Chanel's foam hanging hellishly from her mouth. When they got to the hospital, Chanel was brought in with the nurses lightly slapping her face, telling her to "hang in there, dear". Fortunately, there was a Doctor Brown at the hospital, who was an excellent paediatrician, and he diagnosed her weak muscle illness as Myasthenia Gravis. He ordered an injection of Tensilon,
a drug that would have sent her into cardiac arrest if she didn't suffer Myasthenia Gravis. Chanel responded to the medication and Martin, tears in his voice, told Karla that when Chanel coughed it was sweeter music than a heavenly chorus. He was a strong, burly man and Karla loved him for his sensitivity and almost religious devotion to his family. He told her he was going to night it out at the hospital with Chanel.

Karla said she'd phone his work and tell them he would be taking a leave of absence. After

THE GOLDEN SANDALS

telling his children how much he loved them, Martin told Karla he'd phone them in the morning. When Karla hung up the three of them danced circles, holding hands and laughing while tears of relief and joy escaped their eyes. Then, Karla slowed down the shining times and said she had to make a few calls.

She began by phoning Victor, her father, and told him that Chanel had been diagnosed with Myasthenia Gravis, a disease rarely found in children. He said if she needed anything just to ask. She thanked him and systematically phoned her relatives and friends and told them the news that Martin had relayed: that Chanel had the worst case of this disease attacking a child that Dr. Brown had seen in twenty years. Her brother, Rod, with whom she'd had a special bond since they were toddlers, swore he would help her any way he could. He was a big man like Martin and had two young children himself.

When Karla finished talking to Rod, she told Anne and Burt that they could watch TV on the other couch tonight until they fell asleep. The three of them would be going to the hospital tomorrow Karla told them, but she emphasized getting rest if they were too excited to sleep.

"Will Chanel be having operations, Mom?" asked Anne. It was a good question and very astute of Anne.

"It's too soon to say but let's hope not," she replied as she rose and closed the curtains to the darkness and turned on a bright lamp. The house was peaceful as a lamb now, the dark dragon of Chanel's illness burnt by Dr Brown.

"Do we get to see Chanel and her Doctor Brown?" asked Burt.

"I think so, dear. We'll find out tomorrow. "Karla had almost lost the intimation that they

THE GOLDEN SANDALS

would be getting to know Dr Brown, as her mind had been so preoccupied with her golden-haired angel, Chanel. She wondered what he looked like, whether he was old or young. She thought he must be a genius to save a child, gravely ill, in just a few moments, when many specialists had been puzzled by Chanel's dark and mysterious muscle disease.

Soon, Burt fell asleep and Karla was holding Missy on her lap while talking to Anne. She lit up a smoke and told her daughter that she was a big help looking after Burt when Chanel got sick. And she said that Anne was such a ray of sunshine inside this formerly bleak house, pitching in with cleaning and helping Karla and Martin with meals.

"Anne, dear, I know it's been hard for you with a sick sister and you not getting the time and things you need for yourself. You'll be in high school in the fall and I promise we'll get you started with everything a young girl needs. Like new clothes and other stuff. Grandpa Victor mentioned that he would also see to helping you kids until Chanel is better."

"Thanks, Mom. I love you."

"I love you too, Anne." In a few minutes Anne was asleep and Karla was watching Larry King. She was aware that none of the family had had a goodnight's sleep in the last few months, so she was happy her exhausted children were once again one with the sandman. She smiled to herself and soon fell into a dreamy slumber.

THE GOLDEN SANDALS

Chapter 2

The moon glared like a one-eyed black cat at night. Karla knew the stretch of highway that wound like a tail was going to be a fight for control; yet her car purred along with her big, white cats, Timmy and Missy, sitting behind her in her Mercury Cougar. She liked to take her cats out everywhere - especially when her neighbours had once disapproved of her "two cats in the yard", in their yards. Even tonight beneath the solitary moon's blacktop sky, she was glad they were with her.

She was afraid of going to Chanel's new pad since the brakes on her beloved Mercury Cougar were almost shot, and she had planned on getting them fixed tomorrow, the first day of fall. But as long as she remained cool on the dark road and calculated her speed, she was sure that she, Timmy and Missy would survive. She leaned back on the fur of her headrest, and felt the moon's staring disapproval.

She thought of Chanel as she slowed for a curl in the highway. She had said on the phone that she had heard something scratching at her door. She was alone and Karla knew her "little love kitten" (or "Kit" as she liked to call her) needed her at two AM. Karla would not let her down, as the trees began to lap up the light of the moon. She looked at Timmy and Missy in the rear-view mirror and they both gave her that sleepy, contented look that was characteristic only of cats.

The moon suddenly jumped clear of the trees on an open leg of the highway, almost rewarding her thoughts of Kit's safety instead of her own selfishness. She thought of Kit's great beauty and how Kit used to like to pounce on her as a child, and kiss her awake as Karla catnapped on her new couch. She was impulsive, which had made her purchase the farm forty miles from Karla's place. Karla didn't want them to be apart, but Kit was stubborn about buying the house, barely reading the clauses of the contract when she signed it. But, Karla felt that since it was her dream, she would back her precious daughter who had been so ill.

Karla slowed down just then, her headlights pausing on a road sign. Four kilometres to go. The moonlight licked the road ahead of her car as she stepped up her speed slightly. She was becoming as anxious as a pacing tiger in a cage that'd lost his stripes. She was getting closer to Kit's farm when suddenly, about fifty meters away from her front gates, Karla spotted a large demonic being, screaming that he was going to eat Chanel as he stood before her headlights, directly in her path on the road. She hit the brakes, but they went and her car skidded and slammed into the ditch on the other side of the road. Karla sat, stunned for a minute or so, until Timmy and Missy were growling on her stomach and looking at her with their big, moon cat's eyes to see if she was okay.

Finally, her senses crawled back into her, and she thought about the demonic bear - or whatever it was - and she pawed for the door handle. She opened the door and Timmy and Missy jumped out, their heavy bodies no longer weighing her down. It wasn't long before her two big cats had clawed the eyes out of this death black bear. She got out of the car, still slightly dazed.

Suddenly, Kit was calling her and she looked around to see her young, healthy daughter flying towards her! She dropped into Karla's arms and told her mother the grizzly bear had been trying to get into her house. Karla kissed her as she sobbed that the bear had killed her dogs and small farm animals. They turned towards the grizzly bear's carcass. Karla told her that Timmy and Missy, her two little cougars, had torn the animal to pieces in their powerful catfight. It was dead. Kit

THE GOLDEN SANDALS

began to cry and told Karla that Timmy and Missy were their white Manx cats that had died last spring. Karla looked at the gun in her hand as Timmy and Missy disappeared like ghosts. Her car was in the middle of the road. The moon went behind a cloud and it started to rain, as Karla wondered how she had shot the death bear when she had never even fired a gun. Then, Kit disappeared into the mist and Karla heard a sharp ringing in her ears...

Chapter 3

Karla awoke to the phone ringing on her coffee table. It was Martin. He was at the hospital with Chanel.

"How's Kit?" Karla asked, still half asleep. "Is she okay?"

"Doll, you're dreaming. Who the hell is Kit?" he said, somewhat alarmed. Karla then told him that she'd had a nightmare.

"I'm sorry, hon. I dreamed Chanel was older and well, and that our cats, Timmy and Missy, and I killed a demon bear. But it was dark and horrifying. Is Chanel coming home soon?" She knew she was changing the subject deliberately as she lit up a smoke, noticing Anne and Burt were stirring from the early morning phone call. It was seven-thirty AM.

THE GOLDEN SANDALS

"It's just stress, doll, but it's strange you had a bad dream when Chanel had a good dream that she wants to share. Just a second, Chanel - and...uh...oh, Chanel will be in hospital for probably quite a while. They are putting her on a drug called Mestinon as well as steroids. I'll tell you more later. Here's Chanel, love ya doll."

"Hi, Mom. I love you. I'm sorry you had a bad dream." She sounded stronger to Karla than she had for months. "But Mommy, I had the most wonderful dream. I was sitting in a chair, when a very nice man dressed in white took me to a place where I could walk again. But you know what? It seemed like I was a lot older and I had a farm with little animals and I lived alone, about forty miles from you. And you and Daddy would visit me and we'd ride horses, white ones, and plant vegetables and feed the kittens, lambs and other animals. I even drove a Mercury Cougar and you had one just like it. I had a college degree and I wrote books. I think the farm was where I would like to be someday, and the man in white said he would watch over me like you, Daddy, Burt and Anne do. But you know what, Mommy? Just before I woke up an alien man spoke to me and said I'd get well some day, and that he will always look after me, too. He said the man in white's name was Gabriel."

"That's a very nice dream, punkin', " Karla said, hiding her shock at the common elements of the two dreams. But she thought it was probably just coincidence or, more likely karma. Or even more likely a powerful mother-daughter spiritual bond. Yes, Karla thought, it must be spiritual. Then, it occurred to her that Chanel's dream was about innocence while Karla's was dark and protective - perhaps the killing of the demon-bear symbolized the death of Chanel's illness. She was still perplexed, juggling her emotions about the two dreams, until she finally put the dreams to rest as two journeys intertwined with love.

THE GOLDEN SANDALS

"Are you listening, Mommy?" asked Chanel.

"Oh...uh...yes, sweetie. Would you like to talk to Burt and Anne? They're itching to talk to you. I love you and we'll see you today." She handed Burt the phone. Burt and Anne each talked to Chanel, so Karla hustled into the kitchen to make a quick cup of tea and have a smoke. She was sat at the kitchen table waiting for the kettle to boil, when Burt appeared and sat on her lap.

"What time are we going to see Chanel, Mom?"

"As soon as we can. So have a bath and get clean clothes on." Anne came in after Burt said he would have a bath. He took off with such energy that Karla wished she could transfer some of his zest to Chanel. Anne brought a cup of tea over as Karla looked up at her suddenly.

"Are you okay, Mom? You seem lost in thought. Here, have your tea."

"Thank you, my sweet girl. I'm okay, I was just thinking about Chanel."

"She'll be alright Mom," said Anne. Karla's mood was elevated by the kindness of her daughter. Anne had been forced to grow up fast and had taken care of Burt during the day when Karla was doing things for Chanel. Karla recalled, as she knew Martin did, the days when they'd have to bathe and clothe Chanel, at first thinking Chanel was being lazy and manipulative. The doctors had been unable to find out what was wrong, and Karla now felt the storm of guilt that she and her husband carried because they had both been in denial. She winced with a ripped-up heart at the times when she and Martin had tried to force Chanel to climb the stairs over the last few months.

THE GOLDEN SANDALS

Karla finished her cigarette and tea and decided to make breakfast. She could hear the shower going so she knew Anne was getting cleaned up. By the time Burt and Anne were groomed and dressed, Karla had made the three of them bacon, eggs and toast. They ate their breakfast and then Karla took a long relaxing shower, remembering the days when she and Martin had showered together when they were newlyweds. She was anxious to see how much Chanel had improved and was glad Martin had been there throughout Chanel's terrifying ordeal. She loved Martin as much as she ever had.

Karla dressed and even applied make-up for the first time in several weeks. She looked in the mirror and noticed her eyes were less puffy. Then she phoned Martin's work and fed the cat before they left to see Chanel.

Chapter 4

Karla felt her children's torment passing as she drove to the nearby hospital. She was wonderfully surprised to see her brother Rod's van in the parking lot and told Anne and Burt that Uncle Rod was here to see Chanel. Her eyes spilled tears of pent up grief and Anne asked why she was crying.

"I'm just happy to be with our family since Chanel is getting better. It's okay, I'm not sad anymore." They got out of their Mercury Bobcat and crossed the hospital grounds to the big automatic doors that welcomed them into a world of hope. Karla found Chanel's room on the fourth floor and had to restrain Anne and Burt from racing into the room. As they entered, excitement lit up on everyone's faces and Karla was hugged Chanel with Anne and Burt.

"How's my baby?" Karla asked, as Rod

patted Karla's back and Martin delivered her a kiss that was full of love.

"I feel better, Mommy. I love you! And Anne and Burt!" Karla felt tears hurrying down her face again. Anne's eyes jellied with tears as Karla noticed the huge machines and snaking wires that were hooked up to Chanel's left arm. She had at first thought that Chanel just had IV's and maybe a heart monitor, but these machines looked frightening. She wanted to ask Martin about these metal monsters, but instead mumbled to her husband that she'd phoned the department store where he worked and had arranged a leave of absence for him.

"Speak up, doll," answered Martin, so Karla asked him to go outside so they could discuss Chanel's treatment for the Myasthenia Gravis. Karla and Martin slipped out into the hallway, where he told her that Chanel was being sent to The Vancouver Children's Hospital today. Karla asked her husband if he wanted her to go with Chanel and stay with her until eight PM, then she could take Anne and Burt home. He said yes and he would stay the night with Chanel who was still extremely ill, he emphasized. Karla thanked him with a kiss for she knew he was protecting her from a very disturbing night in a depressing hospital, after he told her Chanel would be there for quite awhile. They decided that one of them would be with Chanel at all times for her reassurance. They hugged and went back into the frightening hospital room.

After everyone had told Chanel how much they loved her and to get well soon, Karla's father Vic walked into the room and was greeted with delightful surprise. He hugged them all and presented Chanel with a stuffed cat and dog - her favourite animals. He asked her how she was feeling and she replied that she was happy and tired. Then, they all turned as a doctor and nurse entered. The former was Doctor Brown and Karla

THE GOLDEN SANDALS

thanked him for saving her daughter's life. When he told them they were transferring Chanel to The Vancouver Children's Hospital now, Karla and Martin informed him of their plans for one of them to be with Chanel at all times. He agreed as he checked the machines and asked Chanel how she was feeling. She said she felt weak; then the nurse gave her some pills and juice. Karla winced inside after seeing her child being dosed with medication. Dr Brown said he would see them at the other hospital in the morning and then he left.

Karla and Chanel hugged their family members' goodbye and prepared for the trip to Vancouver. Vic slipped a hundred dollar bill into Karla's hand and winked as he and the rest of her family were leaving. Karla thanked him. The nurse and other hospital workers began unhooking Chanel's tubes and machines, as Karla held her daughter's hand, reassuring her and smoothing back her child's curly brown hair, that was as long as a horse's mane. She could sense

Chanel's fear and consoled her saying that everything would be okay.

The trip to the children's hospital was agonizingly slow, even by a tortoise's standards Karla thought, but she was relieved when Chanel's eyes began to flutter just as they got there. Chanel was taken to the fourth floor and was asleep by the time the workers and nurses had hooked her up to those sinister machines. Several doctors came in and asked Karla about Chanel's illness and also spoke to her about specialists and interns that would be coming in to see her child. Karla said she'd discuss it with her husband. They did not stay long, and Karla was grateful for Chanel having her own room. She watched her cherub child sleep as her eyes watered, probably smearing her cheeks with mascara. After awhile, she rose and went to the nurse's station and asked where the cafeteria was. Everything was a blur, as she barely remembered eating a ham sandwich in the cafeteria; her thoughts were so

THE GOLDEN SANDALS

filled with Chanel's illness. After eating, she decided to go outside for a smoke to try to relax.

    She went through the main doors and found a bench where she lit up her first smoke in many hours, it seemed. After a puff or two, she noticed a woman of about thirty with dark circles under her eyes that was standing besides her smoking a cigarette. They each said hi.

    "You have a child here, don't you?" The woman asked, almost rhetorically.

    "Yes, a seven year old daughter."

    "Did she just come in today? I haven't seen you around here before, and you have that haggard look that we all have when our children are very ill. I have a five year old son with cancer who has about two weeks to live according to the doctors. Is there hope for your child?"

Greg Bauder

"Yes, she did come in today. She has a rare muscle disease called Myasthenia Gravis. She's going to live but will be in a wheelchair when she gets out of the hospital, the doctors said."

"If you don't mind I'd like to give you a little advice. When I first found out about my son's illness last summer, I was in denial, and then I went through a grieving process which wasn't about death, because at that time there was still hope. But you grieve for the loss and change in the happy, healthy and playful child you once had."

"I didn't know that, but I guess I'll have many hard lessons to learn now that I've got a very ill child. Oh, by the way, I'm Karla."

"I'm Vera. I only wish we didn't have to meet under these circumstances. But my husband, George, is waiting upstairs and I told him and my son that I'd be right back. But I'm sure

THE GOLDEN SANDALS

we'll get to talk again. See ya," she said, as she put out her cigarette butt. Karla watched Vera enter the hospital, and noticed Vera's head and shoulders were slouched as she walked.

Karla sat in silence for another ten minutes and then went back to see if Chanel was awake. On the way from the elevator on the fourth floor, she saw a young couple crying and holding each other in their arms, a doctor and nurse were consoling them. Karla felt sick to her stomach and very dizzy. She knew from their expressions and snippets of conversation that a child had just died. She turned around teary-eyed and realized she was in the cancer ward. She had gone left instead of right from the elevator! She had wandered onto the cancer ward by mistake because of the stress brought on by her daughter's illness.

Karla entered Chanel's room after drying her eyes. Her child was still asleep. She looked lovingly at Chanel, remembering her dancing at two years old to Anne's music, her ringlets bouncing on her back. She had loved to dance. Or when Chanel had dressed up as a bunny for her first Hallowe'en, and Martin had barely kept up with her as she ran from house to house. She thought of her daughter's love of bike-riding, swimming and softball, and the tears leaked out of her eyes.

Karla felt bitter when she considered the hell her child and others went through. How could an all-powerful loving god allow such sweet, innocent children to suffer? Especially, she thought, when He could put an end to it right now. She realized, then, that the universe and God or gods were mysteries that few knew anything about. She vigorously clung to the idea that there were great rewards in the next life for such brave and innocent, suffering children. She thought of Vera's child, and Christ's words: "suffer the little children to come unto Me."

THE GOLDEN SANDALS

Chapter 5

Karla sat by her sleeping Chanel, nursing a coffee. She yawned, and suddenly a wild-eyed, old man sat down beside her. He was pale and small, with a long nose and grey hair, but he had a powerful spiritual and physical presence. He spoke to her, with agony hoarsening his voice. He asked her if he could unburden himself with a confession. Karla said yes, feeling like a strange doctor or priestess, as she glanced at the room's clock. He began after he took a sip of his drink.

"I made a mess of things here on earth. I chose to love people who throw away food and to allow poor children to suffer. And I saw to almost everybody's blindness through my media. I was never really afraid, but I spied on everyone with my finks and cameras. Then, my wrath - one of the seven deadly sins - would come down on those who displeased me."

Greg Bauder

Karla was beginning to shake because she thought this bizarre, black-eyed man was possibly a demon out to test her. So she tested him.

"You know, Shakespeare said: 'The devil can cite scripture for his purpose'. Do you think that's true?" Karla asked, as his eyes looked down into hers and forced her to squirm a bit.

"I know it's true," he responded dolefully. "That's why I'm testing you with this mysterious information. You see I have killed and tortured people and creatures on this planet for centuries. The main reason was because of my bitterness at being alone for so long – and you can't imagine my loneliness - until heaven and earth were created. Then I was forced to try to live up to others' expectations."

They both began to cry. But he continued as a voice from somewhere said, "HURRY UP PLEASE, IT'S TIME."

THE GOLDEN SANDALS

"You see, I tempted Eve because I was celibate... and she was...is so beautiful...and I never knew love so...I...I...I treated women badly." His head and body shook as he sobbed. "When I watched the earth being destroyed there was so...so...much chaos, that I...I...made love to Eve." He put his head in his hands and began to shiver, moaning, "The waste, the waste..."

Then an Angel of Mercy was there putting her arm around his shoulders. She radiated love, and Karla thought that Milton said to her that her daughter's heart was "th' upright heart and pure". She realized then that there was no "usefulness in uselessness" as Chuang Tzu once thought.

"Are you okay, Mr Jehovah? Don't forget that this was your first planet." She smiled at Karla and said, "Karla, I think it's time for Mr Jehovah to get some rest in his hospital room." Karla felt a hand tugging on her sleeve and looked at Chanel's worried face.

"Don't feel bad, Mommy. It was only a dream." She hugged and kissed Chanel with sleep still in her eyes. Karla glanced at her watch. It was five o'clock. She was relieved she'd only had a dream.

THE GOLDEN SANDALS

Chapter 6

Karla watched Chanel fall asleep. She began to remember the horror of Chanel's illness, when her deepest, motherly instincts were screaming at the target of her husband. She realized that both she and Martin had been in denial and their family had been pitted into hell's deepest chasm, especially when they fired words of war around their children. Karla began to cry softly as she thought of the tormented arguments.

She recalled the first signal that something was wrong with Chanel was when Chanel had begun to gain weight. Karla remembered repeatedly discussing this with Martin who also planted seeds of concern because Chanel had been an almost wildly active child. She had been the brightest star on her softball team and yet she gained weight when Karla saw that she was the most active child in the neighbourhood. Karla's thoughts faded as her eyes grew heavy. She noticed that sleep took her into sands of time.

Karla walked The Unknown Desert in the winter wasteland. She called for Gabriel as her feet blistered while carrying her load. She knew the Big Beast was lurking in the beyond preying on the weak. She saw him rising out of her mind, the Big Beast whose baptism of faithful fire had beat on her brow, searing even Eliot's wasteland with its dreaded golden eye. Yet, she knew when the Big Beast wins somewhere the green growth of life is lost, adding strength to the wasteland.

But, the Big Beast began to change its shape into a bird of prey and Karla knew she had to rest. She dropped her burden and fell onto a dune. Her eyes opened as the bird approached and she tried to cry but couldn't. She looked at her burden; a child's bones bleached white, with flies buzzing from above. The Big Beast laughed in the distance in the early morning of the white wasteland world.

THE GOLDEN SANDALS

Karla rose and followed the Big Beast. Her dream was to force him out of The Unknown Desert and into the realms of the river of life and mysticism. She would see him starve with suffering just as he had filled himself with a child.

Suddenly, Karla saw the Big Beast laughing and dragging a woman around by her hair through the wasteland. It was Vera! Karla screamed as she understood that the dead child was Vera's. Karla woke up to her Chanel's touch on her hand.

"It's okay, Mommy," Chanel said. "It's good to cry. That's what the nice man, Gabriel, told me." Karla was perplexed and thought Gabriel must be a doctor's name here.

"I love you sweetie," Karla said. A nurse came in just then so Karla hugged Chanel and left for a smoke. She walked down the despondent halls and caught the elevator. She was surprised to see Vera in the elevator.

Greg Bauder

"Hi, Vera," Karla said. "How are you?" Karla winced as she'd asked a rhetorically ill-conceived question. Vera didn't seem to mind, though.

"I'm about as well as can be under the circumstances, I guess," Vera replied. "How about yourself?"

"Not too bad, considering. Oh...by the way Vera, my daughter is in room 412 in case you want to visit. I understand if you can't but you're welcome to."

"Well of course I can." Vera smiled through her pain. Karla had always been aware of the need for friendship. Her brother Rod had made friends where most people couldn't, and this characteristic had rubbed off on her slightly. That was why her father, Vic, had wanted him to be a politician because of his natural charisma, intelligence and wit. But Rod had always been more satisfied riding his Harley.

Karla felt a hand on her shoulder and knew that Vera was letting her know she had spaced out in thought.

"I'm sorry, Vera. I -"

"Don't apologize, Karla. I've been there and understand."

"Thanks, Vera. If you'd like, maybe I could visit you and your son sometime. I'm already finding that it's good to have support and compassion - as you are letting me know."

"That's right," Vera said with a smile through her agony. Karla noticed how physically beautiful Vera was despite the torture she was going through. Karla knew there was no pain on earth greater than watching your child suffer and die, as you stand helplessly by. The two women puffed on their smokes sadly, yet grateful for company.

    Suddenly, the cloudy Vancouver sky began to unleash rain. The two women put out their cigarettes and ducked back into the hospital. Karla felt the rain added to the gloom and despair to the hospital. She asked Vera if she wanted company to see her son, but Vera said maybe another time. Then, Karla had a revelation as they parted in the halls after hugging each other. Her dream had warned her of the emaciated skeleton child and Vera had protected her from seeing the Big Beast, the personification of Death.

THE GOLDEN SANDALS

Chapter 7

Karla entered the room and saw Chanel was asleep. She looked at her daughter's stressed, haggard face and collapsed in a chair. Then a wave of grief hit her and she fell asleep crying as she recalled a painful memory. She remembered stepping down from the 19 Kingsway bus as its engine buzzed to a complete stop. Somehow she had ceased to be herself and was feeling dead-tired. The once sturdy maple trees hung weakly over the streets as she walked on their crunchy orange-red leaves that had dropped, shaken by a cold, Arctic wind.

It had been October 1977 in Vancouver and Karla had had a feeling it was going to be a rough winter, which was unusual here. Winters in Vancouver usually meant a lot of rain like her sister city, Seattle, about a two-hour drive south. Karla had stopped to look over her shoulder at the snow-topped range of mountains that reigned over the city. They were breathtaking; looking like the ultimate blueberry sundaes. But this picturesque moment had surprisingly turned sour, and only upset her weak stomach into a mini-volcano, as she had held back its avalanche of lunch in her burning throat. She turned away, lifting her legs as though she were in two feet of snow. Why did Mother Nature's beauty suddenly leave her so uptight? Was it something she ate at school maybe? Something was eating at her so she reflected on her day.

Karla was twenty and she had only been to two classes that day at the University of British Columbia: French and Classical Studies. She had wandered lonely, her head in a cloud thinking of the professor's quote of Euripides: "never that which is, shall die". She didn't really believe it. She kicked the leaves and swore at the neighbour's barking pit bull, as she tried to mount a justification for God or the after-life. University professors always sent a wave of new ideas to challenge the

THE GOLDEN SANDALS

"Alps of Science", as Alexander Pope wrote, and progress to them was a burning drive for the student to climb the ropes to higher learning. But today she was stuck in her muddled thoughts.

She thought of her French exam. Normally, she would have been snowed under with only a B grade; after all, she was nearly fluent in French. But something was biting at her mind. Whatever it was had been affecting her studies. She had approached her yard and saw her three sisters in the front window. Strange, she had thought, her older sister from Surrey, a distant Vancouver suburb, there with her two year old daughter, Liza, she noticed. She never came here and Karla barely knew her. Karla entered the house, feeling her heart trying to escape her chest.

"Karla," her youngest sister said, "Mom has cancer." The three were teary-eyed, and Karla dropped her bag and mouth.

"No, no!...No way!" She shouted.

"Yeah, Karla," said her other younger sister, "It's bad. The doctors did an exploratory when she collapsed today. She has bowel cancer. She's in a coma."

The next week was a blur of going to the hospital, going to school and working. Karla was in denial, and thought the entire family was. She lost all faith in life and God as she angrily watched her mom collapse into the rancid jaws of the hungry Big Beast. She was also very pissed off that the doctors were unable to help her mother.

Karla remembered the service for her mother was large, as she was extremely well loved. Her maiden name was Meeks, and she hoped the meek would inherit the earth. If anyone deserved it, she would be the first. But, Karla didn't remember crying at the funeral. She had held a mountain of feelings inside.

THE GOLDEN SANDALS

A few days after her mother's passing on, the entire family gathered at her sister's in Surrey. It was about midnight and they were all talking in the living-room. Suddenly her niece, Liza, came running down the hall screaming. Her mother asked her what was wrong, as her brother-in-law gathered the toddler in his arms.

"I saw Grandma in a brown box...and there were flowers and people...and...I..." sobbed Liza. They settled her down and finally Karla's sister got her back to sleep. Karla thought, as her two brothers did, that she'd simply overheard the adults talking. But her brother-in-law and sister revealed that strange things had been happening with Liza. For one thing, she had an imaginary friend who she would talk to and seemingly wait for him to answer her.

Then, Karla woke up in a sweat as she remembered Liza's "imaginary" friend's name was

Gabriel! She looked at Chanel who was still asleep, and Karla dozed off again.

THE GOLDEN SANDALS

Chapter 8

Karla's snow coloured hands shook like large blossoms in a cool wind. The Big Beast raged in her head telling her to drop the LSD, but she was the Tin Man - she didn't have the heart. She was also off the Valium for the first time in ten years, but she wasn't going to tell anyone. This time she would live dangerously. It was the last straw for her. She had been on tranquilizers and she had prayed and sacrificed herself to God for many years, holding on to a life that would frighten almost anyone. Now, she was going to add to her life with LSD to escape.

Next, she was floating through space, through a dark tunnel and she blacked out. She came to, in a strange wonderland. She guessed that she had asked Alice and gotten her answer. She was in a dim corridor, and she knew she was being observed. Surprisingly, she felt more at peace and more rational than she had been for many years.

But, there was eeriness to those eyes that watched her. She couldn't quite see them but their presence was almost spiritual.

She felt her mind was on display, as she entered a large room with those eyes piercing through glass, watching, carefully distant. They welcomed her and suppressed the voices that once hound-dogged her. She thought of Elvis just then, and he appeared and kissed her. He told her she was in a good place, and then he vanished, leaving her awestruck.

Karla noticed other people there, and they were all in long, bath like robes, of different colours. Her robe was blue. "My favourite colour," she said out loud. Her words became like dreams, free and hard to understand. But, somehow those watching eyes made her go to her room and know that her injection would be soon. She entered her room in a dreamy space. Her room seemed to sink like an elevator dropping slowly.

THE GOLDEN SANDALS

She saw shadows and shapes drifting by her door. Their voices sounded different, yet more real than the strange inkling of the night she...but, she couldn't remember. She heard their words rising, cold and clinical. Laughter echoed in the cool, tense air and she began to shiver. Her thoughts were tagged, as she looked at her wrist knowing those eyes were keeping a calm, collective watch.

She rested on the soft white mattress in her room; there were no other furnishings. A symbol of staying here as time sailed agonizingly into more time, yet somehow she felt it couldn't be forever because it started at a certain point in time. Karla was feeling more alienated than ever, though longing to be free.

"Hi, Mommy," said a familiar voice, and Karla saw Chanel in a pink robe with a man in a white robe. "Don't be afraid. You're on one of Gabriel's spaceships. You will be helped here so you can look after us better on the Earth-Mother."

Karla watched in pleasant surprise as Chanel floated into the room to give her a kiss and hug. She was holding her child telling her she loved her.

After a few minutes it seemed a nurse took Karla to a large hospital type room. Here, a strange voice behind her told her to lie down on a table and not to worry. She was very fascinated by this voice. It said he was a doctor and he was going to give her a needle so she could go home. He came around on her right side and she was shocked to see that he had big, black almond-shaped eyes, and his head was large and light grey. His arms were thin and his three-fingered hands felt rubbery on her forehead. The needle sank into her neck and she cried out, more out of fear than pain at the small, alien doctor's injection.

THE GOLDEN SANDALS

Then Karla woke up to Chanel's touch on her hand. They were in the children's hospital.

"I'm glad the doctor alien helped us Mommy. Look! There goes Gabriel's spaceship!

Karla looked out the window, watching the golden ship arc up high in the morning sky...

Chapter 9

Karla sat amazed as Chanel got up and walked; her daughter was healed. They walked down the hospital hallway as Chanel explained that Gabriel and the little alien doctors had helped her and all sick children. She said not to worry about Vera, and Chanel also knew that someday she would live on a farm as Karla had dreamed. Chanel told her mother Vera's sadness would turn to joy. Just then, Vera approached Karla with a big smile.

"Karla! My son is healed!"

"That's fantastic!" Then both women were shocked as Chanel began to float in the air above them.

"I can fly Mommy," Chanel said. "The alien men use the gravity of the stars to travel and they have given all sick kids the power to float like me

THE GOLDEN SANDALS

and be well."

Karla turned to hear a large commotion as all the kids in the ward were floating. The nurses and doctors were wide-eyed and still. Chanel said God had seen enough suffering of children. She said flying was a gift only for sick kids.

The next day, Karla brought Chanel home and the newspapers and TV were full of the news that the ill children were healed and could fly. Her family had gathered at Karla's and they knew a new era had begun in the world.

WOOFED COOKIES by Greg Bauder

Little Christy Madison lived in a big chocolate coloured house; except for the window sills and doors, which were white, like vanilla ice-cream. Christy and her two best friends, Betty and Amos, called it the gingerbread house. Christy felt proud and happy to live in such a nice house with her mother, Dolly, and her father, Ken.

But today Christy was sad as she sat on the bed in her pink room. Her blue eyes shone with tears above her pouting mouth. Here she was, she thought, eight years old today and her parents had not bought her a puppy. It was her biggest dream and if her parents wouldn't buy her one, then she wouldn't want them to throw her a party. Instead, she would stay in her room.

There was a knock on the door.

"Christy, you need to come downstairs now," said her mother gingerly. "The party's going to be starting."

"I 'm not going to my birthday party!" Christy almost shouted. Her mother entered the room. She, like Christy, was very pretty with blonde hair and natural ringlets.

"Is it because you don't think you'll be getting

THE GOLDEN SANDALS

a puppy?" her mother asked.

"Yes, " said Christy.

"Well, you never know dear," answered her mother. "But as Daddy and I have always told you, puppies need a lot of care and are hard to look after. But come to the party, okay?"

Christy's eyes lit up and she bounced up off the bed.

"You mean I might get one? Okay, I'll come down." They walked out of Christy's room past the lace-white curtains in the hallway windows that she liked to call the coconut curtains. They walked down the winding stairs and entered the lemon coloured kitchen. Christy's family and friends began to sing 'Happy Birthday'. Her two aunts and her cousin, Chip, were there; so were Betty and Amos. Then she saw her cake and the presents on the table; it was a puppy cake, but there was no real puppy! She was almost ready to cry, when suddenly her Dad whispered behind her "woof, woof ". She turned around to see her father holding a small, grey puppy in one hand.

"Happy Birthday, sweetie," he said, and she hugged him and everyone else. Then she held the little puppy in her hands and patted him.

"This is the best present I ever had!" she squealed with joy and tears of love for the little puppy. She held it next to her ruby cheeks. "He looks like Dorothy's Toto from 'The Wizard of Oz!' I love him!" After she patted, kissed and loved the little puppy for awhile, her father put the little dog into a box so Christy could blow out the candles on her cake and open her presents.

"I'm not going to wish for anything because my wish has come true," she laughed, and blew out the candles on the cake. Then, she opened her presents which she liked; but even the Barbie

THE GOLDEN SANDALS

doll she got wasn't near to her heart like the little grey puppy. After Christy thanked everyone for the gifts her mother cut the cake.

"Can my puppy have a piece?" asked Christy, her blue eyes bouncing bright.

"Christy, do you know how you feel if you eat too much cake or ice-cream, or if you have the flu? You feel sick. So don't give the puppy cake or he'll get sick and woof," her father said gently.

"Okay," said Christy. They ate Oreo ice-cream, followed by some cake. After a lot of 'Happy Birthdays' from her family and friends they left and Christy begged her parents to let her keep the puppy in her room in its box. They said it would be okay.

She took the puppy into her room and put on her pyjamas, while watching with love the little grey puppy trying to jump out of the box. She picked him up and got into bed. She patted her little dog's paws; he was panting and playful.

"Are you hungry?" she said, thinking that he was begging for food. She had a box of Animal Cracker cookies on her night table. She thought these would be okay for the puppy because of their name, but she would only give him two because she remembered what her father had said about cake and ice-cream.

The little dog ate the tiny Animal Crackers greedily and then begged and whined for more. But Christy was afraid to give him too many, so she cuddled him and turned out the lamp, trying to get him to sleep. She began to yawn and feel sleepy as the puppy snuggled up to her neck.

She awoke to a frightening yapping, just as the light came on in her room. Her parents were there and the little puppy was throwing upon her pink comforter.

THE GOLDEN SANDALS

"Did you give him any cookies?" asked her father.

"Just Animal Crackers, Daddy."

"Well, now he's woofed his cookies."

"What does that mean?" asked Christy, scared.

"It means he threw up, Christy," said her mother gently.

"Remember Christy, you should never give puppies sugary things like cake or cookies," her father said. "But don't worry, he'll be okay." The puppy was at the foot of the bed where the light brown stains were. He was shivering slightly as Christy's dad put him in the box.

"I see, Daddy. So he won't woof his

cookies. You know what? I think I'm going to call him Cookie!"

MY WRITING CAREER by Greg Bauder

Recently, I have considered writing a book about my life's experiences. I had pondered about it before but wrote it off my mind because I'm not too good at writing comedies. Or in this case, a comedy of errors. If I did though, I'm sure it would be the next generation's chief source of inspiration - er, I mean perspiration - if they ever tried reading and understanding it. I've always heard that good writing is mostly perspiration, anyway. In that case, a book from me would be no sweat.

It's true that most great epics begin in the middle like Milton's PARADISE LOST, although Byron did his DON JUAN from the beginning, of course. So I guess to subvert these traditions that means that I'll have to start at the very end. Well, the end is nowhere in sight - so much for my epic. But, if I could start at the end it would be a novel approach, I think. So, instead, how about some little cameos from my smoking, writing career.

The first story I remember writing was in grade four. It was a jovial tale about a trip to Jupiter in a spaceship. (Some may say I didn't have enough literary sense to stay away from Science Fiction even then!) I recall describing a friendly monster there as being ten feet tall. The teacher asked me in big, red letters on my marked story if I measured the monster in it. This was my first painful introduction to (gulp!) criticism.

I also remember writing in high school a piece about a drug deal, loosely based on my own experiences. Like Wordsworth's "memory recollected in tranquillity", the drugs I took then, and the prescribed ones that I take now, are supposed to keep me tranquil. But, the story was a bust and only introduced me to writer's cramp. Marking my words was easy: I didn't say much.

Greg Bauder

In my early years of college, the extent of my creative writing was mostly poetry, and even that was limited. There was no reason and a lot of rhyme for it. My professors willingly suspended their belief that I could write. (Yes, I know Coleridge's exact quote - it's not my reading that's in question here). Had Pope read some of my more "meaningful" poems, he probably would have written a sequel to THE DUNCIAD about me.

Now, I think the word is finally out on my writing (or lack thereof). My only advice to you is that if you're reading this somewhere, cancel your subscription immediately!

THE GOLDEN SANDALS

EDUCATING FRED by Greg Bauder

I smile when remembering Fred's negativity towards university.

"Never bothered with it," Fred said. "All talk; sitting in chairs ain't tough stuff." Fred felt that a college education was baloney. He seemed, to blue collar workers, the epitome of toughness and had recently been promoted foreman at a big mill. His fingers and hands were covered with thick, hard scars. "Ever work eight straight hours like our men get to do? Well, hell if it ever occurred to you to do so, go apply at our workplace. Enough of this silly college nonsense."

"But what," I replied, "about accountants, doctors, lawyers, architects, engineers? In addition, we'd be living in shit without advanced mathematics." I eyed his grin, showing missing teeth he had probably once bashed in scrapping.

Greg Bauder

"We need some of course. Your degree means peanuts because it's English Literature. We read whatever interests us. Fussy lecturing professors teach Shakespeare; I like Mickey Spillane."

"Do you realize," I answered, "words represent the steps of us gaining understanding? Every writer with skill has a portion of history he must fulfil. Love of choice, voice and a Miltonic polemic gave America free speech. Writing like Milton did revolutionised Western thinking; his thoughts brought religious tolerance; his writing justified divorce; his insight turned clergymen's corruption public; and, one of his manifestos averted Church support for government control. In addition, Milton's pen had a hand in supporting Cromwell's disempowering of the English King."

"Shut up! What bunch of malarkey bull was that! A writer like this Milton guy died many years ago. No way Jose, can man be freed by writers."

THE GOLDEN SANDALS

"How about the Bible? Moses wrote some of it, didn't he? We are part of the biblical influence. Moses freed his people. Writers like Milton, Virgil and Atwood feed readers new views that affect us. Thus, it is clear we need reading habits that evoke the growth of the intellect." Fred's countenance softened; I realized I might have had a vast influence with his thinking.

"Maybe there is something in this college knowledge. But fuck, man! Can I sign up?"

"Yup," I replied. Fred graduated three years ago with distinction, at England's Cambridge University.

Greg Bauder

REGRESSION by Greg Bauder

Buzz in your head

What does it mean? Slowly you come to. You live in a psychiatric
boarding home.

Med-time now bed-time over

You slowly roll out of bed. You slip into your housecoat.

Open door focus mind

You stagger slightly down the hallway; sleep is falling from your
eyes.

Line-up shift feet

Today you're meeting a friend. You tell the nurse

THE GOLDEN SANDALS

as you swallow pills.

Retreat to room voices faint

You get dressed and groomed for the day. It's been awhile since you
looked forward to meeting someone this much.

Chore mops bathroom floors

You tell the activity worker you've done your chore. You won't be back
for an hour or so. It's nine o'clock.

Sign board slip out door

Your friend has his own place. But you're meeting him at the restaurant.

Footsteps follow on sidewalk

Finally, the restaurant door looms. You go inside.

Greg Bauder

Friendly wave sees
you.

Sit down tea for two

You pour the tea he'd ordered and ask him how he's been.

Depression rules even wise men

You tell him you're doing well. Medication has cleared up voices.

Satan's voices torment souls

He's glad the voices are subsiding. He says he was suicidal up until a
week ago. He looks tired.

Meds hindered his thoughts

But you respond by saying meds help a lot of

THE GOLDEN SANDALS

mentally ill people.

Voices visions are handicaps

He disagrees. Then, he tells you a secret after you promise not to disclose
it.

He offed meds this week

Intrigued, you ask him what differences he's noticed.

His spirit flies high

You ask him to tell you exactly what he means.

Spirit beamed into shiny wheel

Into a spaceship? You ask him enthusiastically.
He nods.

Greg Bauder

Free and just universe

He tells you that spiritual growth is vital in our many lives.

Pills pull you down

He states that he has seen wonderful places and has become more mature spiritually.

Angelic nature verified by many

You know this. Everybody likes him and his company and his wisdom.

God's aliens deliver safely back

You ask him what they look like. You hope they coincide with your past
visions.

Jehovah rules Pleiades angels

THE GOLDEN SANDALS

Angels are golden people. God is more mysterious and different, he says. He will not tell you how.

Fly away together tonight

He says it's possible. But much would be expected of you. He would rather see you continue with writing.

Popped balloon destiny

He quotes The Bible: "Blessed are they who have not seen and yet have believed." He says it's from John 20:29.

Bible proof of truth

He says the Apocrypha and Gnostic Gospels and other holy texts are just as valid in God's eyes.

Greg Bauder

Hard understanding foreign beliefs

To be with Jesus, safe and sound, that is your goal, you say.

Love goodness and faith he says

You agree. You ask him if he would like to come back to the boarding home. He used to live there.

Hope falls to earth

He says no but will visit you in a dream tonight and will take you on a journey through your past.

Shock ignites belief

You ask if he'll be in a spaceship. He states that it will only be a spiritual journey.

Filled with thrill

THE GOLDEN SANDALS

He says much of your past will be painful as his was. But he has been charged with the mission of setting your soul free.

Enthusiasm spills over you

It may take many years, he says. It all depends on you.

Mysterious mystic hope

He says he will concentrate on your present life. He claims that you have lived in Sumerian, Mayan and Atlantan cultures just as he has.

Wisdom derives from experience

But some people never seem to learn, you say. He agrees.

Spiritually immature repeat scenarios

Greg Bauder

You must go now, he states. He will meet you tonight when you least expect him. Eventually, you will find that you no longer need pills.

Hug mystic priest

You leave, wondering why more information wasn't exchanged. You decide to throw meds away, too, as you leave the restaurant.

Walk in clouded thoughts

You arrive back at the boarding home. You lay down until it's time for lunch.

Lunch blurs by mind

You rinse your dishes, then line up for meds. The nurse hands you your pills.

Mouth pills turn quickly

THE GOLDEN SANDALS

You walk down the hallway. No one can see you as you put your pills deep into the garbage bag inside the garbage can.

Goodbye thrill to pills

You go into your room and lie down. Your thoughts race.

Wonder about friend's words

You drift off to sleep and awake at the five o'clock shout for dinner. Dazed, you leave your room and go to the dining-room.

Food gobbled scarcely tasted

There seems to be more tension in the air than usual. You squirm uncomfortably in your seat until your table is excused.

Dishes cleaned ready for wash

Greg Bauder

You line up for dinner meds. More Haldol. The nurse asks you how you are feeling.

Okay you mouth pills

You walk down the hallway and palm the pills deep into the garbage again.

Fly free tonight hopefully

You go to your room. But you are restless and can't lie down and be still.

Pill withdrawal necessary

It's a stage you think. Your friend is a very trustworthy person.

Rise turn on radio

The steady beat comes in waves. Softly, it plays

THE GOLDEN SANDALS

the music.

Pace to pleasurable sound

Finally, after several hours of vegetating about music, you turn the radio off and head for the living room.

Horseplay in mad swing

You never involve yourself in these games. The nurses are always telling the younger guys in the boarding home to stop play-fighting.

Wrestlers trip over your feet

You tell them to be careful as you gaze at the TV. You can't seem to follow what's on.

Wait for med-time

Finally, the nurse announces that it's time for

medication.

She eyes you intently

You didn't have a snack at 8 o'clock tonight, she noticed. Plus, you seem agitated she observes. Do you need to talk?

Negative as you mouth pills

You turn away to place pills in the garbage bag, again.

Pace halls 'til bedtime

It's 11 o'clock. You get undressed and jump into bed with your heart jumping with excitement.

Gradually drift to sleep

Then, your friend appears to you in a white robe through the window. You rise and find yourself

THE GOLDEN SANDALS

passing through the wall and window.

Peacefulness surrounds your friend

Suddenly, you're observing a boy on a raft, sinking fast.

Repeat of childhood trauma

He is you. You are saved by an older boy who plunged into the river to rescue you. You remember the incident from childhood.

Friend asks how you feel

You're frightened, but somehow you know that it was not your time to die then.

You fear death by water

Then, you are tuned in to another scenario. This time you are cutting through a neighbour's yard on

Greg Bauder

the way home from elementary school.

Guard dog attacks

The dog lunges for your throat but the chain sends him careening backwards. The chain had stopped the dog's jaws inches from your throat.

Shaken reminded of fear

Your friend turns to you and asks what you've learned. Other people's privacy is as important as yours, you say.

Many possible reasons for dog

He nods and tells you you're learning, but tonight is just a baby step.

Always patterns in things

You do not understand that fully. Next, you are

THE GOLDEN SANDALS

watching yourself freaking out on LSD at the age of fifteen.

Your teen spirit rose disembodied

You are terrified. You do not want to think of this. Then, the truth hits you, you think.

From water to animal to human

You've evolved on a spiritual trail that is parallel to, but much lesser than, God's evolutionary scale.

Your friend agrees beaming

Suddenly, you are back on your bed crying and shouting, begging for your friend to come back.

Nurse enters your room

She wants you to come to the office. You follow her there and she tells you to sit down. An ambulance arrives.

Incoherence blurs reality

You vaguely remember the hospital ride to the emergency room.

Hospital bed night

Channels flow through your TV mind. Mostly cartoons as you lay there.

Control is lost freely

Childhood nightmares haunt your stationary pillowed head.

Advertise your need for help

A nurse announces herself with a flashlight. You tell her of cartoon shows.

THE GOLDEN SANDALS

Voices bug the bunny

She does not understand.

Donald drinks Mickey under the table

You tell her you're mad at the world. Alfred E. Neumann needs to be punched out.

Spiderman spins web of deceit

Superman is green around the gills because of Kryptonite, you say. The nurse leaves and returns with liquid Haldol. You swallow it.

Robin has gone batty

Bats in his belfry, like you. The nurse says try to get some sleep.

Underdog is sinister Simon says

Then, you realize the cartoons are part of your childhood experiences when you felt more secure. But they have mixed with psychotic anger and confusion.

Feel daffy as a duck

Somehow, you finally fall asleep and wake up in the hospital. You consider telling the nurses and doctors you went off your meds.

Lessons learned regardless

You sigh as you get out of bed and leave the room. You have decided you need your meds as you join the line up. You hold out your hand.

www.ingramcontent.com/pod-product-compliance
Ingram Content Group UK Ltd.
Pitfield, Milton Keynes, MK11 3LW, UK
UKHW041412180426
11947UKWH00007B/73